Understanding

Urology

Making Urology Endoscopy 'EZ'

José A. Claudio Bonilla

Dedication

To you, dear reader,

Thank you for allowing me the opportunity to share my urology experience with you. Within these pages, you will find - or perhaps refresh your memory with - knowledge of various urology procedures, the equipment and supplies needed for a range of endoscopic urology procedures, how these procedures are performed, and more. My thirty-eight years of urology experience is now in your hands. I encourage you to diligently obtain the necessary equipment and supplies based on the procedure at hand, and to apply the innovative techniques outlined here.

I hope and pray that this knowledge supports you on your journey!

- José A. Claudio Bonilla

Acknowledgment

My passion for urology began amidst the surgical fluids, urine, and blood that would cover the operating room floor. It started with the distinctive smell of burning tissue - an odor few would ever want to experience. But it also began with my desire to learn, grow, and share the knowledge I've gained over the years.

There was a time when disposable urology packs didn't exist; everything was reusable clothes and linens. There were no fluid pressure bags, cameras, monitors, flexible ureteroscopes, or lasers. Ureteroscopy was done without scopes, and stones in the kidney or ureter were removed using baskets, often blindly, hoping the stone was engaged. Open surgeries for large stone extractions were common.

Innovation has been a cornerstone of urology's evolution, and I've been fortunate to witness and contribute to these advancements. Many urologists have welcomed my insights, valuing my voice and presence in the operating room. With this acknowledgment, I honor those who have invested their time, talents, and resources to help shape me into the surgical technologist I am today.

I honor the memory of Dr. Manuel Fernando Alsina Capó (1909-2008), known to our Tito Mattey de Yauco Operating Room Team in the 1980s as "Alsina Capó." He was the co-founder and President of the Asociación de Urólogos de Puerto Rico in 1957.

I proudly exalt the memory of Dattatraya G. "Datta" Wagle, M.D., FACS (June 29, 1936 – January 24, 2020) - the first physician from Western New York to head the American Urology Association. At St. Joseph Catholic Health System in Buffalo, New York, our team performed around thirty procedures every Monday and Friday. My presence during his cases, especially during open nephrectomies, seemed to give him confidence. He would often say, "José, please call my office and let them know the days you are off so I won't schedule any open cases." Rest in peace, Dr. Wagle.[1]

---

[1] Buffalo News. (n.d.). *Dr. Datta G. Wagle, 83, first Western New York physician to head American Urological Association.* Buffalo News.

I also cannot forget the incredible urology team at Mayo Clinic Hospital - where I was once a member - and the urology surgeons, especially Dr. David D. Thiel, M.D., former Chair of the Department of Urology and Director of Robotic Surgery at Mayo Clinic Hospital in Jacksonville, Florida. Dr. Thiel, with an open mind and trust, allowed me to introduce innovative practices into the Mayo Clinic urology team, where my input was always welcomed.

Now, at Ascension Riverside in Jacksonville, Florida, I continue to share my time, knowledge, energy, and resources. I want to recognize our 'Green Team' of nurses, techs, and surgeons. Among them, I honor Dr. Julia Han, MD, who has given me the confidence to express my innovative knowledge during ureteroscopy and other endoscopic procedures; Dr. Richard Lewis, Co-Director of the Stone Prevention Program and Director of the Prostate Cryosurgery Program; and Dr. Hayden Hill, MD, who has welcomed my input during robotic

----

https://buffalonews.com/news/local/dr-datta-g-wagle-83-first-western-new-york-physician-to-head-american-urological-association

surgeries.

> *"José has genuine appreciation and dedication to the field of urology. With over thirty years of experience as a surgical technician, he has a diverse and rich set of surgical skills and knowledge base. Whenever we operate together, he shares how the particular surgery was done in the past and compares its evolution to current day practices. He is able to give first hand testimony on how surgical approaches and technology has evolved which speaks to the innovation in the field of urology."*

\- Dr. Julia Han, MD (Monday, August 19th, 2024).

About the Author

José A. Claudio Bonilla is a Surgical Technologist with a Master of Divinity (M.Div.) and a Master's in TESOL. He shares his life experience in urology with *Making Urology Endoscopy Easy 'EZ'*. In addition to being a writer, José is a pastor, preacher, speaker, singer, teacher, surgical technologist, and baseball player. Above all, he is deeply passionate about social justice and Christian religious education. His commitment to social justice began during his time as a Community Organizer at the Gamaliel Foundation in Chicago, Illinois, and his passion for Christian education was underpinned during his time at Colgate Crozer Divinity School in Rochester, New York.

José has been actively involved in public advocacy, championing causes such as better education, improved transportation, and fair immigration laws, among other pressing social issues. Born in Puerto Rico, where he took his first steps in the operating room, he later lived in Western New York, where his focus on urology grew, and now resides in Northeastern Florida, where he continues his work in the field. Throughout his journey, José has shown deep compassion for patients with urological conditions, believing that education, preparation, and provision are some of the most important things in providing the best care, with the patient always being the top priority in the operating room.

José began his surgical technology education in Ponce, Puerto Rico, in August 1985, and is proud to have served as the surgical technologist for Dr. Manuel Fernando Alsina Capó (1909–2008), co-founder and President of the Asociación de Urólogos de Puerto Rico in 1957. He also worked alongside Dr. Dattatraya G. 'Datta' Wagle, M.D. (1936–2020), the first physician from Western New York to head the American Urology Association. Additionally, José worked at Mayo Clinic Hospital in Jacksonville, Florida, with the urology team led by Dr. David Thiel, M.D., former Chair of the Department of Urology and Director of Robotic Surgery.

Now, as a Preceptor at Ascension Riverside in Jacksonville, Florida, José continues his work with the hospital's 'Green Team,' one of the operating room groups. José continues to share his time, energy, knowledge, and resources with others, striving to make a difference in the lives of his patients and colleagues.

Table of Contents

Introduction

Welcome to an exciting urology journey full of insights, understanding, and stories designed to simplify your urology practice, build your confidence, and help you practice fearlessly.

Hola! My name is Jose A. Claudio Bonilla, and I am a Urology Technologist with 38 years of experience in the field. My motto, "I love urology," reflects my dedication, which was strengthened during my time working at one of the world-renowned hospitals in Northeastern Florida. I am passionate about urology and am here to make it as easy ("EZ") for you as possible!

Since 1986, immediately after graduating as an Operating Room Technician, I have been occupied with urology and its challenges. These challenges demand an experienced team with the knowledge, skills, and competence to work confidently without the fear of not meeting the doctor's needs. Such fear can lead to frustration, anxiety, and even feelings of rejection from colleagues. Imagine a surgeon requesting something that isn't readily available or within reach, or envision yourself as a circulating nurse constantly running in and out of the room to fetch items for the surgeon. This situation often occurs during urology procedures, especially when they are performed outside of the dedicated urology suite.

That's the reason that the main goal of my writing is to provide you with insights into urology, help you prepare for procedures, and enable you to anticipate the surgeon's needs while performing those procedures. I want to highlight this clearly: "There is no 'routine' in urology!" Urology, particularly cysto-ureteroscopy, is based heavily on findings even before the scope is introduced into the bladder through the urinary orifice. It is very important for operating room personnel to stay attentive to what the surgeon is doing, has done, and will do. In other words, your experience in the field will greatly contribute to successful teamwork.

Before I conclude this introduction, I would like you to keep in mind some of my sayings:

- "Keep the fluid flowing."
- "Be prepared and anticipate" - have different options ready.

- "Have it available" - keep items close to you, not in a room next door.
- "Wait to open it" - only open items when needed to avoid shortages of instruments or supplies.

These sayings can help you maintain a clear understanding of the surgeon's actions, prevent excessive bleeding and visibility issues, and expedite the procedure. They also help avoid anxiety, frustration, and communication problems, among other potential issues.

Understanding Urology Procedural Terminology

Since urology is the main focus, the terms or abbreviations used here describe various urology procedures. Here are some of the most common ones:

- Cyst: A sac containing fluid.

- Oscopy: Visualization using a lens, scope, or camera.

- Retro: Backward, behind.

- Litho: Stone.

- Pexy: Fixation or attachment.

- Paxy: Crushing and extracting.

- Lapa: Abdominal cavity.

- Raphy: Suturing.

- Uretero: Ureter.

- Urethro: Urethra.

- Tripsy: Breaking up or crushing.

- Nephro: Kidney.

- Trans: Throughout.

- Uro: Urinary tract.

- Lift: Lift or hold up.

- HoLEP: Holmium Laser Enucleation of the Prostate.

- HoLAP: Holmium Laser Ablation of the Prostate.

- Supra: Superior.

- Ectomy: Removal.

- Otomy: Cutting.

- Ostomy: Creation of a drainage cavity.

- Circ: Around.

Now, let's combine some of these terms with body anatomy to describe common urology procedures:

General Terms

1. *Cyst*oscopy: Visual examination of the bladder using a cystoscope. This instrument allows the surgeon to examine the urethra, prostate, and the lining of the bladder, as well as other related areas.

2. Urethr*oscopy*: Visual examination of the urethra.

3. UTI: Urinary Tract Infection.

4. *Retro*grade: An imaging test that uses X-rays in a *backward* motion during a cystoscopy procedure.

5. Urolithiasis *(uro-lithi-asis)*: Presence of stones in the urinary system.

6. *Cyst*ogram: X-ray of the bladder using a catheter and contrast material.

7. Ureter*oscopy*: Visual examination of the ureter, the duct through which urine passes from the kidney to the bladder.

8. Ureteral Stent Placement/Extraction: Placement involves inserting a thin, hollow tube into the ureter to help urine flow from the kidney to the bladder. Extraction involves removing this tube.

9. Stone Manipulation/Lithotripsy: The process of extracting or pulverizing stones from the kidney, ureter, or bladder.

10. Ureteral Calculi: Stones located in the ureter.

11. Laser *Nephrolithotripsy*: Pulverizing and extracting stones located in the kidney using a laser.

12. Cystolitholapaxy: Crushing and extraction of bladder stones.

13. *Ureteroscopy* Using Dual Laser for Ureteronephrotic Tumors: Visualization of the ureter and kidney while treating tumors with a laser.

14. UPJ (Ureteropelvic Junction): The area where the ureter connects to the kidney pelvis.

15. UBJ (Ureteral Bladder Junction): The area where the ureter connects to the bladder.

16. Uretrocele: A sac or dilation of the terminal portion of the ureter.

17. TURBT (Transurethral Resection of Bladder Tumors): A procedure for removing tumors from the bladder using a transurethral approach.

18. TURP (Transurethral Resection of the Prostate): A procedure for removing part of the prostate using a transurethral approach.

19. TUIP (Transurethral Incision of the Prostate): An incision made in the prostate, often including an incision of the bladder neck.

20. UroLift: The lifting or expansion of the urinary tract in the prostate using a special UroLift disposable lift applier, a 2mm cystoscope, obturator, and cysto sheath. Some doctors may use a flexible cystoscope for an initial examination before using the UroLift application instrumentation.

21. Clots Evacuation: Removal of blood clots (hematuria) from the bladder.

22. Botox Injection: Insertion of a cystoscope into the bladder to inject Botox into multiple sites via a needle that fits through the cystoscope.

23. Bulkamid Injection: A procedure involving the injection of Bulkamid, a gel used to treat urinary incontinence.

24. Green/Red Light Laser Therapy: Heating and vaporization of excess prostate tissue using green or red light lasers.

25. HoLEP (Holmium Laser Enucleation of the Prostate): A procedure that uses a holmium laser to remove prostate tissue.

26. HoLAP (Holmium Laser Ablation of the Prostate): A procedure that uses a holmium laser to ablate (destroy) prostate tissue.

27. Suprapubic Tube Insertion: Creation of a channel from the skin into the bladder to insert a urinary tube.

28. ESWL (Extracorporeal Shock Wave Lithotripsy): A non-invasive procedure that uses shock waves to break up kidney stones into smaller pieces.

Prostate Biopsy or Space OAR Related

1. Transrectal: Performed through the rectum. A prostate biopsy involves removing tissue samples from the prostate using a thin needle inserted through the rectum, sometimes with the aid of an ultrasound probe.

2. Transperineal: Performed through the perineal space. A prostate biopsy involves removing tissue samples from the prostate using a thin needle inserted through the perineal area (the space between the anus and the scrotum), often guided by an ultrasound probe.

3. Gold Seeds or Space OAR: Using an ultrasound probe, gold seeds are inserted into the prostate through the perineal area with a slightly larger needle than that used for a prostate biopsy.

Scrotal or Inguinal Related

1. Male Circumcision: Surgical removal of the skin covering the tip of the penis.

2. Hydrocelectomy: Removal of a fluid-filled sac adjacent to the testicles.

3. Orchiectomy: Surgical removal of one or both testicles. This can be performed through the scrotal or inguinal approach.

4. Orchiopexy: Surgical repair or attachment of a testicle to the scrotum with a tacking stitch.

5. Varicocelectomy: Surgical removal of dilated or enlarged veins along the spermatic cord.

6. Vasectomy: Surgical procedure to cut and seal the vas deferens, which carries sperm from the testicles.

7. Vasectomy Reversal (Vasovasostomy): Surgical repair of the vas deferens to restore fertility.

8. Urethroplasty: Surgical repair of the urethra.

9. Artificial Urinary Sphincter (AUS) Placement: Placement of an AUS through an incision in the perineum and a small incision in the abdomen.

10. Urodynamics: Diagnostic examination of bladder and urethral sphincter function.

11. Penile Implant and Prosthesis: Artificial devices placed inside the penis to allow men with erectile dysfunction to achieve an erection.

12. Penile Plication: Surgical procedure to correct penile curvature.

13. Puvo Vaginal Sling: Synthetic sling (hammock-like) device placed under the urethra and attached to the abdominal wall to prevent urine leakage.

14. Cystocele: Bladder herniation into the vaginal canal.

15. Vesicovaginal Fistula: Abnormal passage between the bladder and vagina.

16. Marshall Marchetti: Abdominal procedure to address bladder control issues or incontinence.

Abdominal Related:

1. Open Prostatectomy: Removal of the prostate gland through an abdominal incision.

2. Open Cystectomy: Removal of the bladder through an abdominal incision.

3. Open Ureteroplasty: Surgical repair of the ureter.

4. Open Total/Radical Nephrectomy: Total removal of a kidney through a thoracoabdominal or abdominal incision.

5. Open Partial Nephrectomy: Partial removal of a kidney through a thoracoabdominal or abdominal incision.

6. Open Nephroureterectomy: Total removal of a kidney and ureter through a thoracoabdominal or abdominal incision.

Robotic/Laparoscopy Related:

1. Laparoscopy: Visualization of internal abdominal organs using a scope.

2. Robotic Prostatectomy: Robotic-assisted removal of the prostate gland.

3. Robotic Cystectomy: Robotic-assisted removal of the bladder.

4. Robotic Ureteroplasty: Robotic-assisted repair of the ureter.

5. Robotic Total/Radical Nephrectomy: Robotic-assisted total removal of a kidney.

6. Robotic Partial Nephrectomy: Robotic-assisted partial removal of a kidney.

7. Robotic Nephroureterectomy: Robotic-assisted total removal of a kidney and ureter.

Back Related:

1. InterStim: Implantable device that sends mild electrical pulses to stimulate the sacral nerves.

Equipment and Supplies Needed for The Following Procedures

In this section, we'll focus on how to select the case, prepare the operating room, and gather all the necessary equipment and supplies for a successful procedure. Let's approach each case one at a time and work as a thoughtful team. Before diving into the details of each case, let's first consider the following table, which outlines the continuous fluid flow used in various cystoscopy/ urology procedures:

Procedure	Fluid	Comment
Cystoscopy	Water	Some urologists prefer N/S.
Cystoscopy stent placement, stent exchange	Water	No need to use N/S.

Cystoscopy ureteroscopy (diagnostic, stone lithotripsy, and tumor ablation)	N/S	Fluid must be pressurized (raise the fluid, use a pressure bag, or install a pressure device, such as a single-action pump system). If monopolar coagulation, such as Bugbee, is used, switch N/S to water and apply pressure.
Cystolitholapaxy	Water	-
TURBT, TURP, and TUIP	Water, N/S, or Glysine (for TURP only, if preferred by the doctor)	It depends! Water for monopolar, N/S for bipolar. Continuous flow N/S irrigation may be used at the end of the case through a three-way Foley.
Greenlight laser ablation of the prostate	Water and/or N/S	Some surgeons prefer to start with water and then switch to N/S. If this happens, remove the water bag from the irrigation system to

		avoid confusion. Continuous flow N/S irrigation may be used at the end of the case through a three-way Foley.
Cystoscopy Botox or Bulkamid injection	Water	-
Nephrolithotomy	N/S	No pressure is needed, though some surgeons prefer a pressure bag or system for the entire case. If a ureteroscope is used, a pressure bag, cysto tubing, and stopcock may be required.
Holmium laser enucleation of the prostate (HoLEP) and Holmium laser ablation of the prostate (HoLAP)	N/S	Continuous flow N/S irrigation may be used at the end of the case through a three-way Foley.
Urolift	Water	-
Suprapubic of a	Water	Have it ready in case

catheter drainage		a cystoscopy is performed.
	17	

Cystoscopy

Let's make it "EZ" by calling this setup the 'default table.' It's called default because, no matter what the surgeon is doing, if a lens is being inserted into the bladder, a cystoscopy setup is needed. In other words, for every cystoscopic case, regardless of the specific procedure, we'll prepare a 'cysto table' (the default setup) and then add whatever is necessary if additional procedures are involved. For example, if the surgeon is placing a stent, set up the 'default table' and add contrast, an open-ended catheter, a guidewire, and the actual stent, if needed. Be sure to follow the doctor's preference card.

Now, let's put the 'default table' together. Assume the case is set up as follows:

- Cysto pack

- Cysto tubing (if not included in the pack)

- Cysto drape (if not included in the pack)

- Doctor's gown

- Doctor's gloves

- Cysto instrument set

- Cysto camera

- Cysto lenses (30° and 70°, 4mm)

- Lubricant gel and/or uro-jet 2% lidocaine

<u>Cystoscopy Set Content (30° and 70° Lenses May Be Separate):</u>

- 17, 21, 22, and 25 Fr. sheaths (may be in the set). A simple cystoscopy may be done with the first three. The 22 Fr. is typically preferred by many urologists (color-coded).

- One obturator for each sheath size (17, 21, 22, and 25).

- Short bridges (x2): one single lumen, one double - the majority of urologists prefer the single lumen.

- Rubber caps (x2) for placement on the short bridge lumens.

- 30° and 70° cysto lenses (may be kept separate from the cysto set).

- It's wise to include a hemostat and scissors in the cysto set or have them available separately.

- Waterport for fluid tubing control.

- Flexible grasper, specifically for use with the rigid cystoscopy set (not the flexible scope).

- Albarran bridge (optional).

- Light cord (sometimes kept with the cystoscopy instruments, separately or with the camera).

<u>Organizing the Procedure Table (the Default Table):</u>

Arrange the table as efficiently as possible, paying close attention to where the surgeon prefers the items to be placed. Many urologists have specific preferences for table setup. This means making the gown and gloves visible to the surgeon; positioning the legging and cysto drape on one corner of the table; placing containers and fluids on another corner; making sure the camera, light cord, and fluid tubing are visible; organizing the cysto instruments with the 30° and 70° lenses; and using a towel or a 4x4 sponge to hold the lubricant gel. Once all these items are on the table, they are ready for use, and your default table setup is complete (Figure #2).

Take the following instruments from the cysto set:

- 22 Fr. sheath (the blue one).

- Single lumen short bridge (some surgeons may prefer the dual lumen one).

- Rubber cap (place it on the short bridge).

- 30-degree cystoscope (the one with the red band).

These are the initial instruments needed to begin the cystoscopy procedure. They can be assembled together or laid out visibly for the surgeon. With these items prepared, the default table should be all set!

Notes:

1. Make sure the cystoscopes have the correct and compatible light cord connectors.

2. Add the camera and light cord to the default table if needed.

3. Include water and/or N/S, omnipaque (if needed), uro-jet, and/or jelly lubricant.

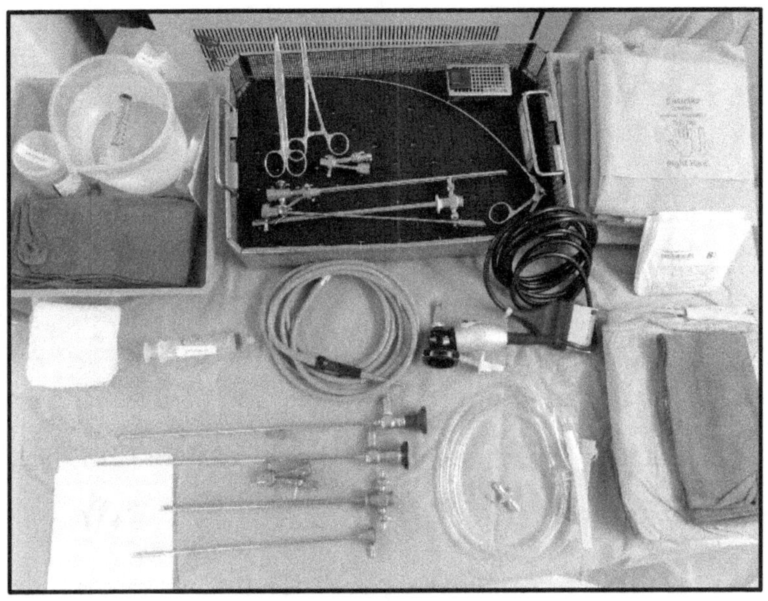

Basic Equipment, Monitors, and Other Essentials

Let's make sure we have the basic equipment ready to perform the procedures. Keep in mind that the following list does not include the equipment, medication, and supplies needed by the anesthesia team. Here's the checklist:

1. Camera source and monitor for each scope to be used (cysto cart). *Note: cystoscopes and ureteroscopes may require different camera sources.*

2. Light source (which may come with different tip insertion shapes and forms).

3. Stirrups.

4. IV pole to hang the procedure's continuous irrigating fluid.

5. Does the cysto cart have a functioning picture-taking and printing feature? Make sure it's operational!

6. If using a flexible cystoscope, ureteroscope, or any other scope, confirm they have compatible camera and light sources (see notes above) and confirm they are working.

7. X-ray table availability: If a C-arm will be used, confirm that the case will be performed in a room with an X-ray table. If not, communicate with the X-ray personnel to have one ready. Is there an electrical outlet for a laser? If so, plug it in and have the laser key available in case it needs to be used.

8. Bovie unit and other energy generators are needed for the procedure, such as monopolar and bipolar generators.

9. Sequential Compression Device (SCD).

10. Procedure set up tables and other necessary furniture.

11. Check if there's enough fluid in the warmer (water, N/S, and glycine).

12. If the procedure requires special instrumentation or equipment not available at the facility, make the necessary arrangements ahead of time.

13. Other items as needed.

Cystoscopy With the Flexible Cystoscope

If the surgeon requests the use of a flexible cystoscope, nothing changes with the setup. Simply add the flexible cystoscope to the default setup. Make sure the following accessories are readily available in case the procedure evolves into more than a simple cystoscopy:

- Flexible biopsy forceps (specifically designed for flexible cystoscopes)

- Flexible grasper (specifically designed for flexible cystoscopes)

- Bugbee electrode

- Bugbee cord

- A piece of telfa

- Hypodermic needle (for removing biopsy tissue from the grasper)

- Formalin containers

- Open-ended catheter

- Guidewire

- Contrast

- Surgical gel or uro-jet 2% lidocaine

26

Cystoscopy and Retrograde or/and Stent Placement/Exchange

For this case, the surgeon will examine the bladder, inject contrast into the ureter and kidney, and, if needed, place a J-stent, remove the old one, or insert a new one. This can be unilateral or bilateral. Therefore, let's set up the 'default table' and add the following items:

- Open-ended catheter (yellow or tigger tail - check the surgeon's preference)

- Guidewire (verify the type the surgeon prefers, such as sensor wire, stiff glide, Benson, or another type)

- Contrast (for X-ray visualization - check if the surgeon prefers it diluted with water or normal saline, and at what concentration - pure, 50/50, or other)

- For stent exchange or placement, make sure there is a grasper compatible with the urology set you are using and according to the surgeon's preference.

- Remember to have 20cc and 10cc syringes for injecting the contrast as well as rubber caps for the cystoscopy set's 'short bridge.'

- Make sure the availability of ionizing radiation protection such as lead aprons, thyroid shields, and personal radiation dosimeters.

Cystoscopy with Cystogram

A cystogram may be performed for various reasons, such as measuring bladder capacity, checking for perforations, or other diagnostic purposes. It can be done by injecting contrast into the bladder either through the cystoscope or using a Foley catheter. This procedure is often carried out alongside other cystoscopic procedures, particularly during bladder tumor resection. Therefore, confirm the following items are available in addition to the default table setup:

- Contrast

- Foley catheter

- 10cc syringe

- Surgical gel

- A piston or catheter tip syringe or a Toomey syringe

- Measuring bowl

- Ionizing radiation protection (lead aprons, thyroid shields, personal radiation dosimeters) whenever X-rays are in use.

Cystoscopy Botox Injection

Botox injections are used to partially paralyze the bladder, helping to reduce urinary urgency and incontinence. This procedure is performed through a cystoscopy, where the healthcare provider assesses the inside of the bladder. There are two key considerations for the team to ensure proper preparation:

1. Botox Units: Determine how many units the healthcare provider will use (100, 200, or 300).

2. Instrumentation, Equipment, and Supplies: Ensure the cystoscopy setup is complete (default table, appropriate injection needle, and fulgurating supplies if needed).

Now, let's get ready to prepare the botox:

1. Botox: Confirm the number of units required. Gather injectable normal saline, 10cc syringes, and hypodermic needles according to the healthcare provider's preference.

2. Needle: Select the appropriate needle for the bladder injection. The 'Sidekick Rigid Needle' is commonly used.

Now, let's prepare the cystoscopy table:

- Set up the default table.

- Include the injectable agent (Botox).

- Add the SideKick Needle.

- Have a Bugbee electrode and cord ready in case of bleeding during injections.

- Make sure the patient is properly grounded.

- Use water for the irrigation tubing.

Notes:

- Set the bovie unit to '0' for cutting and '30' for coagulation (or as per the doctor's preference). Always confirm the settings with the healthcare provider.

- Place the foot pedal within easy reach of the surgeon.

Cystoscopy Bulkamid Injection

A Bulkamid injection is a minimally invasive treatment for stress urinary incontinence (unwanted and involuntary leakage of urine). This procedure involves injecting a bulking agent (Bulkamid) into the urethra to add volume (bulk) to the tissue. The injection is performed through a cystoscopy to visualize the urethra during the procedure.

Therefore, the following setup is needed:

- Default table

- Bulkamid Scope

- Bulkamid Agent (includes the scope sheath, agent, and needles)

- Bugbee electrode and cord (ready in case of bleeding during the injections)

- Make sure the patient is properly grounded

- Use water for the irrigation tubing

Notes:

- Set the bovie unit to '0' for cutting and '30' for coagulation. Always confirm the settings with the healthcare provider.

- Don't forget the foot pedal!

Cystoscopy Bladder Hydrodistension

What Is It?

The healthcare provider fills the patient's bladder with fluid (water or normal saline), sometimes multiple times. It's generally recommended to use water, as it allows for coagulation in case bleeding occurs, which is a possibility. The procedure is used to investigate the causes of bladder pain.

How Is It Done?

The procedure is performed under anesthesia through a cystoscopy. The bladder is filled either via a cystoscope or a Foley catheter. The goal is to fill the bladder as much as possible to determine its capacity. The fluid is then drained, typically into a measuring container, to assess the bladder's full capacity. This process may be repeated, with the bladder being refilled and drained for measurement. A final cystoscopy allows the healthcare provider to examine the bladder lining for any abnormalities or sores related to the patient's symptoms.

Now, let's get ready for the procedure:

- Set up the default table

- Hang a 3000 ml water bag (the healthcare provider may ask for the exact amount in the bag before filling the bladder)

- Have at least a 1000 ml capacity measuring container

- Make sure the following are available:

  1. Various sizes of 5cc Foley catheters

  2. 10cc syringes

  3. Extra water bags

  4. Bugbee electrode and cord

  5. A Foley or leg bag (not commonly used but may be requested)

Urethroscopy

Whenever a cystoscopy is performed via the urethra, the procedure inherently involves urethroscopy, which visualizes the urethra (the tube responsible for draining urine from the bladder out of the body.) It's important to understand the reason for the urethroscopy and whether the patient is male, female, or transgender. These factors help the surgical team properly prepare for the procedure.

Let's brainstorm and organize the setup while preparing for the procedure:

- Set up the default table.

- Lens considerations: Have a 0-degree lens available in the room for straightforward visualization.

- Resectoscope sheath: Have a smaller size, such as a 17Fr., along with various dilator options (for male and female patients), guide wire (according to the surgeon's preference), balloon dilators with pressure gauges, biopsy forceps, and retrieving baskets.

- Contrast: Make sure contrast is in the room and the patient's information is entered into the X-ray system.

- Additional tools: Have a Transurethral Resection of the Prostate (TUR), Direct Vision Internal Urethrotome (DVIU), and cold knife urethrotome ready.

- Stricture concerns: If urethral stricture is suspected, a semi-rigid ureteroscope may also be useful - keep it nearby.

- Filiforms and followers: Make sure you know where these instruments are located.

- Surgical gel: Have an adequate supply on hand.

- Foley catheter: The patient may leave the operating room with a Foley catheter. Have various options available, especially ones with Council tips.

- Foley or leg bag: Make sure these items are ready for use.

A urethroscopy may be performed due to simple urethral irritation, microscopic or gross hematuria, or urinary urgency and frequency. However, it can also address more complex issues, such as urethral strictures or lesions.

Ureteroscopy

There are three main types of ureteroscopy procedures: diagnostic, lithotripsy for stone extraction, and tumor ablation. Although the setup may look similar, the instrumentation, equipment, and supplies may vary. Let's break down each procedure, keeping in mind the necessary items to have nearby or in the room.

Diagnostic Ureteroscopy

Start by preparing the default table. Check with the surgeon before opening the open-ended catheter, guide wire, and contrast, as some prefer not to waste supplies. Have the following items available:

- A second wire (surgeon's preference)

- Flexible ureteroscope

- Semi-rigid ureteroscope

- Various sizes of access sheaths

- Dual lumen catheter

- Pressurized normal saline or manual pump devices (like a pathfinder or slip-tip syringe)

- Ureteral dilator devices (e.g., Nottingham dilator)

- 1.9 stone extraction basket, N-gage, or the doctor's preferred one

- 200 and 365-micron diameter laser fiber (don't forget the laser key, as it may be requested)

- Different sizes of J-stents

- Picture-taking camera system

- Other necessary items

These items should help in making sure that the case runs smoothly.

Ureteroscopy Laser Lithotripsy

Before the procedure, it's helpful to gather the following information:

- Patient's gender

- Whether the patient has been previously stented

- Stone location (proximal to the kidney or distal in the ureter)

- Patient height and weight

This information helps the team anticipate the surgeon's needs for access sheath length, ureteroscope, laser fiber size, and stent size. With this in mind, prepare as follows:

- Set up the default table.

- Add contrast, an open-ended catheter, and a guide wire (based on the surgeon's preference card).

- Have the same items and equipment ready for the diagnostic ureteroscopy.

Nurses and techs should monitor the cystoscopy fluid and pressure bag (if used) to ensure a clear monitor picture, prevent bubbles, and manage bleeding. In many cases, the surgeon may request the stone be sent as a specimen, and hospital policy often requires the stent to be sent to pathology.

Ureteroscopy Tumor Ablation

This procedure is slightly different from diagnostic ureteroscopy or ureteroscopy with laser/stone extraction. Prepare similarly, but make sure the following items are available:

- Normal saline irrigation and water (labeled in different containers) on the default table

- One or two extra 10cc syringes

- Two ureteral open-ended catheters

- Biopsy forceps (1.9-3.0 Fr.) compatible with flexible and semi-rigid ureteroscopes

- Hypodermic needle (to help collect the specimen from the biopsy forceps)

- Piece of telfa (for biopsy samples, if preferred by the surgeon)

- Bugbee cord and electrode (no higher than 3.0 Fr.)

- Brush (up to 3.0 Fr.) for specimen collection

- 1.9/Zero tip Nitinol stone retrieval basket

- Potassium-titanyl-phosphate (KTP) laser (if provided by a sales representative)

- Holmium laser (for tumor ablation)

- 200 or 272 and 365-micron diameter holmium laser fiber

- Specimen cup with formalin

- 20cc syringe for aspirating tumor or kidney fluid for samples

- Sterile specimen cup for urine samples

Notes:

1. Set the Bugbee unit at 0 cutting and 10-20 coagulation.

2. Normal saline is used for ureteroscopy, but if Bugbee coagulation is required, switch to water for better current conductivity.

3. Ground the patient and place the foot pedal by the surgeon's feet.

4. Consider using a pressure pump system like the pathfinder to assist with fluid management.

5. Communicate with the pathology department if you have questions about specimens.

Using KTP Laser For Ureteroscopy

When using a KTP Laser (Potassium Titanyl Phosphate Crystal), make sure the following equipment and supplies are ready:

1. Laser safety protocols: Follow all laser safety regulations, including:

    - Posting laser signs on doors.

    - Providing goggles at the entrance for anyone entering the room.

    - Covering windows.

- Making sure everyone in the room, including the patient, is wearing goggles.

- Having at least 1000 ml of water on the default table.

- Following additional hospital-specific laser regulations.

2. Assistance with the KTP laser: If the facility does not have a KTP laser, assist the laser representative in setting up the unit and help find an appropriate location for it in the room.

3. KTP laser fiber: Make sure that a 200 or 272 fiber is available. Note that higher fiber numbers can compromise the ureteroscope, hinder the irrigation system, and result in a blurry image on the monitor.

4. Laser fiber holding device: Have either a laser fiber holding device or a wet towel ready for use.

5. Laser pedal: The laser representative will position the laser pedal near the surgeon's foot.

Notes:

- Even if a KTP laser is being used, ground the patient in case the surgeon decides to switch to a Bugbee electrode. If that happens, switch from saline irrigation to water, provide the Bugbee cord, ensure the patient is grounded, and position the monopolar unit foot pedal by the surgeon's feet.

- Keep biopsy forceps, the Bugbee electrode, and the Bugbee cord nearby.

- If the Bugbee is used, confirm with the surgeon that the monopolar unit is set at approximately 0 for cutting and 10-20 for coagulation.

- Be creative and proactive in anticipating needs!

Pubic Tube Insertion

This procedure involves the placement of a Foley catheter into the urinary bladder via the suprapubic region, specifically, the pubic symphysis. It is performed on individuals who cannot drain their bladder through the urethra or to replace a urethral catheter with a suprapubic drainage system. It is extremely important for the surgical team to have all the necessary equipment and supplies prepared and ready for use. The following list may assist in preparation:

6. Set up the standard cystoscopy table.

7. Add the following items to the table:

- 20 or 22-gauge spinal needle

- #11 blade with knife handle

- One-Step Suprapubic Introducer 17 cm/20 French (Fr)

- 16 Fr Foley catheter with a 5cc balloon

- 10cc syringe

- Foley bag

- 2-0 silk, nylon, or the suture preferred by the medical provider on a cutting needle

- Suture kit (needle driver, Adson forceps, and scissors)

- Water

Since this procedure can vary, some surgeons may simplify it or choose to insert a larger catheter (such as 22 Fr) using a curved instrument like the Lowsley or Randall (stone extraction instruments). Here's a simplified approach:

- Prepare as you would for the standard suprapubic procedure, but do not open the 'One-Step Suprapubic Introducer 17 cm/20 Fr' unless needed. The spinal needle may also not be required.

- Confirm with the surgeon which Foley size will be used (typically 20, 22, or larger).

- Add a heavy suture, such as #1 or #2 Prolene (just tie), to pull the catheter from the outside of the abdominal wall into the bladder and through the penile orifice.

The concept is to insert the Lowsley or Randall

instrument into the urethra, guide it to the bladder, and push the curved instrument toward the inner abdominal wall near the pubic region. Once the surgeon sees a lump in the pubic area, they will make an incision in the pubic/abdominal wall with the #11 blade, push the instrument through the abdominal wall to expose it, tie the Foley tip to the curved instrument with the heavy suture, and pull the Foley through the penis. After the Foley exits the penis, the surgeon will cut the suture, remove the curved instrument, retract the Foley into the bladder, inflate the balloon with 10cc of water, and test it. Finally, the Foley bag will be attached to the catheter.

Most often, the surgeon will perform a cystoscopy and fill the bladder with fluid (water or normal saline) before conducting this suprapubic catheter insertion technique.

Cryotherapy or Cryoablation

This treatment for prostate cancer involves freezing prostate tissue to destroy cancer cells using a cryoablation system, also known as Visual Ice. During the procedure, thin metal needles or probes are inserted through the perineal space into the prostate, guided by an ultrasound rectal probe and a precision grid. The needles are filled with argon gas, which causes the targeted prostate tissue to freeze.

The operating room will need to be equipped with the following items:

- The operating table

- Camera and light cord-monitor system

- IV pole for cystoscopy tubing and normal saline for the warmer endo-fluid system

- Small table for the warmer unit and fluid pump system (provided by a cryoablation representative)

- Visual Ice Cryoablation unit (provided by the sales representative)

- Two argon gas tanks

- Ultrasound system and monitor

- Ultrasound probe and stepper

- Default table

- Mayo stand

- Anesthesia machine and related equipment

- Small table for clean items, including piston or catheter tip syringe with ultrasound gel, 10cc and 60cc syringes, ultrasound probe, condom, 4x4 sponges, towels, a bowl of water, and other necessary items

- Default table (make sure there is space available when the cryoablation representative provides the needles. Have something heavy on hand to place on top of the needles to prevent them from falling on the floor)

As you can see above, the room is fully equipped. Now, let's prepare for the case:

- Set up the default table as usual.

- Add a few hemostats, scissors, a knife handle, and a needle driver to the default table (a suture may be added if requested by the surgeon).

- Add a 16 or 18 Fr. Foley catheter with a leg or Foley bag.

- Include extra surgical gloves for the surgeon.

- Drape a Mayo stand and place the following items on it: a flexible cystoscope, a guide wire (based on the doctor's preference), a suprapubic spike, a second 16 Fr. Foley catheter (5cc), a #11 or #15 blade, a 10cc syringe with water, a #22 spinal needle, and anything else you think might be useful.

A sales representative will provide a penis insertion warmer, which will remain with the patient from before the procedure begins until just before the patient leaves the operating room or as requested by the surgeon.

The procedure will likely proceed as follows:

- After the time-out, the surgeon will perform a cystoscopy through the urethra to examine the bladder and locate the spinal needle in the suprapubic space before puncturing the abdominal wall with the suprapubic spike.

- Once the spike is inserted, a #16 Foley catheter will be placed through the spiked opening.

- To create space in the perineal area, the surgeon may use staples, a towel, or another tool to hold the scrotum away from the rectum, facilitating the insertion of the ultrasound probe into the rectum.

- After the perineal space is created, the surgeon will insert the ultrasound probe into the rectum.

- With the ultrasound probe in place, the surgeon will insert frozen needles through the perineal area using an ultrasound stepper and a #17 precision grid (the number of needles is determined by the urologist).

- Once the needles are inserted, and just before freezing the lesion, a fluid warmer probe will be inserted into the bladder through the urethra and will remain in place until the patient leaves the room.

- At the end of the procedure, the patient will leave the room with a suprapubic Foley catheter and a leg or Foley bag.

<u>*Note:*</u>

Make sure that all equipment and supplies are available and functional before the patient enters the operating room. This includes having a #14-17 ultrasound grid.

Transrectal, Transperineal Biopsies, and Gold Seeds Space OAR

Transrectal and Transperineal Biopsy

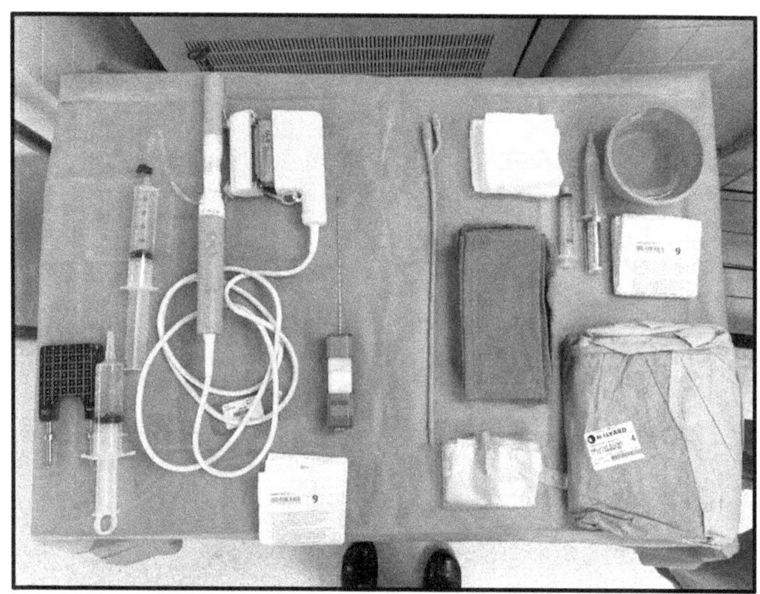

When discussing the 'grid' in the previous section, it's worth pausing to explain some strategies for transrectal and transperineal prostate biopsy, as well as gold seed SpaceOAR placement. Although these procedures are considered clean, maintaining sterile techniques as much as possible is important. Let's separate the clean and sterile fields with two small tables. Additionally, since surgeons often decide to perform a cystoscopy, we'll include a possible 'default' table setup.

<u>Table One - The Clean Table</u>

- Use a table cover.

- Sterile gloves and gown for the surgeon.

- Two packs of 4x4 sterile gauze.

- A piece of Telfa.

- A pack of blue towels.

- Two bowls.

- Water.

- One 60cc syringe.

- One 10cc syringe.

- 1-inch silk tape (6 inches long).

- Six packs of ultrasound gel.

- Inflating condom or a regular condom.

- Biopsy needle (per doctor's preference).

- Transperineal biopsy grid.

- Piston syringe.

- A transperineal ultrasound probe (per doctor's preference).

Notes:

To prevent bubbles in the inflatable condom, follow this preparation process:

- Open a pack of ultrasound gel into one of the bowls and mix it with 5cc of water.

- Draw the mixed gel into the 10cc syringe.

- Wipe any excess gel off the outside of the syringe with a blue towel.

- Insert the syringe into the inflatable condom and inject the gel forcefully to make sure it goes deep into the condom.

- Insert the ultrasound probe into the condom as far as possible and secure it with 1-inch silk tape.

- Fill the 60cc syringe with water.

- Attach the syringe to the condom and inflate it with 10-15cc of water while holding the tip of the ultrasound probe inside the condom. Tap the condom gently to remove any air bubbles, repeating this 3 to 4 times until no more bubbles are visible.

- Place the prepared ultrasound probe on the clean table or the operating room table setup.

Table Two – The Possible Default Table

Open a table cover and include:

1. The surgeon's gloves.

2. A pack of 4x4 sterile gauze.

3. A 10cc syringe.

4. A bowl with water.

5. A Foley catheter and leg or Foley bag (some surgeons prefer a red rubber catheter).

Note:

If the surgeon decides to perform a cystoscopy, add the items listed on the default table.

Transperineal Ultrasound, Gold Seeds, and SpaceOAR

The technique for placing gold seeds and SpaceOAR is similar to preparing for a transperineal or transrectal biopsy. The key difference is the addition of gold seeds and the SpaceOAR, which should only be opened upon the surgeon's request, as they are expensive. Open them one at a time - gold seeds first, then SpaceOAR when requested. Typically, no specimens (biopsies) are collected, and there's usually no cystoscopy or catheter insertion, but a red rubber catheter might be inserted. Be sure to have it ready.

Prostate biopsies can be performed in three ways: transperineal, transrectal, or strictly guided with specialized ultrasound equipment. While the preparation is largely the same, anesthesia varies - these procedures can be done without any (which may be painful for the patient), with local anesthesia, sedation, or under general anesthesia. They can be performed either in the doctor's office or in a hospital setting, on a patient stretcher via transrectal approach, or on the operating room table using the 'Precision Point' technique, one of the newest methods on the market. The setup, however, remains the same.

Don't be afraid! One of the important things is to have basic knowledge and understanding to provide satisfactory care and service.

Transurethral Resection of Prostate (TURP)

TURP is a procedure used to remove part of the prostate gland in men. Since the prostate is located between the penis and the bladder, surrounding the urethra (which carries urine from the bladder to the penis), the procedure is performed through the urethra using electrical energy, either monopolar or bipolar.

There are three main ways to perform this procedure:

- Using monopolar instruments.

- Using monopolar instrumentation with a bipolar working element.

- Using a bipolar loop or oval button plasma system for resection and vaporization in saline.

Using Monopolar Instrumentation

Let's organize the case using monopolar instrumentation. Here's what we need for the TURP procedure:

- A patient grounding pad (required for monopolar current; use a current-conductive fluid such as water, sorbitol, or glycine).

- TURP instruments (monopolar).

- TURP bovie cord.

- Van Buren sounds (sizes 12-34).

- Surgical gel.

- Monopolar loop (24, 27, or 28).

- A Toomey syringe or Elic evacuator.

- Foley catheter (doctor's preference – typically 3-way, 30cc balloon, 22Fr. or 24Fr.).

- 10cc, 20cc, and/or 30cc syringes.

- Catheter guide.

- Urine bag.

- Catheter strap (to secure the Foley catheter to the patient's leg).

- 3,000 ml glycine or sorbitol (ensure 10-12 bags are in the warmer).

- Fluid connecting tube (to use with multiple fluid bags).

- Specimen container with formalin.

- A spoon.

Now, let's set up the operating room. Start by preparing the default table, then add the following:

- TURP instruments (monopolar).

- TURP bovie cord (may be included with the TURP set).

- Van Buren sounds (sizes 12-34, have them available).

- Surgical gel.

- Monopolar loop (24, 27, or 28).

- Toomey syringe or Elic evacuator.

- Foley catheter (doctor's preference – typically 3-way, 30cc balloon, 22Fr. or 24Fr.).

- 10cc, 20cc, and/or 30cc syringes.

- Urine bag.

<u>*Notes:*</u>

- If you're a nurse, don't forget to ground the patient.

- Place the monopolar energy generator foot pedal where the surgeon prefers.

- Start the procedure with at least 2 bags of glycine or sorbitol (use the extension/connecting tube to run two bags simultaneously).

- While the surgeon is working, monitor the fluid closely.

- As the case nears completion, bring 2 to 4 bags of 3000 ml normal saline into the room for continuous bladder irrigation (CBI) while the patient is being transported and remains in the recovery room.

- The monopolar energy generator setting for a TURP should be around 120 for cutting and 80 for coagulation. For a TURBT, the settings should be around 100 for cutting and 70 for coagulation.

TURP Using Monopolar Instruments with a Bipolar Working Element

This approach is similar, with a few differences:

- No patient grounding pad is needed (though keep one available).

- Use normal saline instead of glycine or sorbitol.

- Use an energy generator specifically designed for bipolar use.

- Use the bipolar working element and bovie cord.

- Use a bipolar resecting loop (verify with the sales representative which one is appropriate for the TURP).

- At the end of the case, ensure there is enough normal saline for CBI.

TURP Using Bipolar Loop/Button Plasma System

The procedure is performed with the same intention and in a similar manner as when using monopolar energy. However, this time, we'll organize the case using bipolar energy. Let's gather everything we need:

- No grounding pad is needed in this case (bipolar energy does not require one).

- 3000 ml normal saline (no water or glycine) – 10-12 bags, possibly more.

- Plasma system energy generator.

- Bipolar TURP instruments (e.g., Button TURP).

- Bipolar TURP loop and/or button.

- Van Buren sounds (sizes 12-34).

- Surgical gel.

- A Toomey syringe or Elic evacuator.

- Foley catheter (doctor's preference – 3-way, 30cc balloon, 22Fr. or 24Fr.).

- 10cc, 20cc, and/or 30cc syringes.

- Catheter guide.

- Urine bag.

- Catheter strap (to secure the Foley catheter to the patient's leg).

- Fluid connecting tube (to connect multiple fluid bags).

- Specimen container with formalin.

- A spoon.

Now, let's set up the operating room. Start by preparing the default table and add the following:

- Bipolar TURP instruments.

- Bipolar TURP loop (e.g., the Button).

- Van Buren sounds (sizes 12-34 – have them available).

- Surgical gel.

- Toomey syringe or Elic evacuator.

- Foley catheter (doctor's preference – typically 3-way, 30cc balloon, 22Fr. or 24Fr.).

- 10cc, 20cc, and/or 30cc syringes.

- Urine bag.

<u>*Notes:*</u>

- Begin the procedure with at least two 3000 ml bags of normal saline (use the extension/connecting tube to run two bags simultaneously).

- While the surgeon is working, closely monitor the fluid levels.

- Most bipolar energy generators come with pre-set settings for TURBT and TURP. Please follow the manufacturer's instructions.

- The optimal settings for the energy generator are 200, 120, and TP3. The plasma 'oval button' doesn't require different settings.

- Make sure the foot pedal is positioned where the surgeon prefers.

- As the procedure nears completion, have 2-4 additional bags of 3000 ml normal saline ready for continuous bladder irrigation (CBI) while the patient is transported and during their stay in the recovery room.

67

Transurethral Resection of Bladder Tumor (TURBT)

Bladder tumors (cancer that begins in the bladder) require a setup similar to TURP procedures. The instrumentation and fluids are almost identical, with the exception of glycine and the size/shape of the resectoscope sheath and cutting loop. Glycine is not used for bladder tumors, but it may be necessary if the surgeon decides to resect prostate tissue in men, though glycine is strictly for prostate tissue. To summarize: water and grounding pad for monopolar, and normal saline for bipolar energy.

Since bladder cancer can vary in size and location, the surgical team should prepare for a range of possibilities. A TURBT may evolve into a small bladder biopsy or vice versa. Therefore, it is wise to prepare as follows:

- Prepare the default table.

- Make sure the following are available:

1. Photography Setup: Ensure the urology camera system is ready for imaging (this is very important). Verify that the camera printer has paper and is functioning properly.

2. Biopsy Forceps: Have both rigid and flexible biopsy forceps available (appropriate for the cystoscopy set) to collect specimens (often more than one).

3. If using a flexible cystoscope, make sure the appropriate biopsy forceps for the scope are available.

4. Ground the patient.

5. Bugbee fiber and Bugbee cord.

6. Telfa pads or formalin containers for specimen collection.

7. A 22-gauge needle to assist with removing small samples from the biopsy forceps.

8. A monopolar energy generator (confirm the preferred settings with the surgeon).

9. Position the foot pedal near the surgeon's feet.

10. Make sure there is water and normal saline on the default table.

11. Hang water if using the Bugbee for coagulation.

12. Set the cutting setting on the energy generator to '0' to avoid bladder perforation.

If Monopolar Resection with A Cutting Loop Is Used:

1. TUR tray.

2. #24 loop.

3. Monopolar cord (if not in the tray).

4. A spoon.

5. Make sure there is enough water available, and keep an eye on the levels. Don't wait until the last minute to add more.

6. Have urethral dilators nearby.

7. Make sure the foot pedal is placed near the surgeon's feet.

If Bipolar with A Monopolar TUR Set (Resectoscope Sheath) Is Used:

1. Use the bipolar working element.

2. Hang normal saline or switch from water to saline.

3. Add the bipolar loop appropriate for bladder tumors (verify with the surgeon before opening).

4. Bipolar cord.

5. A spoon.

6. Have multiple formalin containers available.

7. Don't forget the foot pedal near the surgeon's feet.

If the Plasma Cutting Loop and Button are Used:

1. Switch to the plasma energy generator.

2. Use the Button TUR set.

3. Add the loop and cord (as requested by the surgeon) and have the button readily available.

4. Hang normal saline.

5. A spoon.

6. Have formalin containers ready.

7. Make sure the foot pedal is in place near the surgeon's feet.

Notes:

1. Be prepared for any unexpected changes during the procedure and ready to be creative to anticipate the surgeon's needs!

2. The settings for the Bugbee vary based on surgeon preference (commonly 0 for cutting and 20 for

coagulation, though some prefer up to 60 for coag). Always set cutting to '0' to avoid accidents.

3. Monopolar resection settings: 100 cut, 70 coag.

4. Bipolar settings (used with the monopolar resectoscope sheath) are typically pre-set by the manufacturer or representative.

5. Plasma energy settings: 180 cut, 100 coag.

6. Make sure Foley catheters and supplies for continuous bladder irrigation (CBI) are available, along with a Foley or leg bag.

7. Have contrast, a guide wire, and a #5 open-ended catheter on hand (based on surgeon preference).

8. This procedure presents many possibilities, so it's important for the team to stay innovative and adaptable.

Using KTP Laser For Bladder Tumor (With The 3 Options Above)

When a KTP Laser (Potassium Titanyl Phosphate Crystal) is used for bladder tumor resection, make sure that the following equipment, supplies, and regulations are in place:

Laser Setup and Safety Regulations

Follow all laser safety regulations:

- Place laser signs on the doors.

- Provide laser goggles by the doors for those entering and ensure goggles are worn inside by all staff and the patient.

- Cover windows to prevent light leakage.

- Keep at least 1000 ml of water on the default table.

- Comply with hospital-specific laser regulations.

Required Equipment & Supplies

- #17 resectoscope sheath or laser sheath.

- Laser fiber (200, 400, or 600 micron).

- Greenlight scope or a lens filter (provided by the laser sales representative).

- Foley catheter (as per the surgeon's preference).

- Foley catheter or leg bag.

- Toomey syringe.

- A laser guide catheter or open-ended catheter (such as Tigger Tail).

- Laser fiber holding device or a wet towel.

Notes and Additional Considerations:

1. Ground the patient even if the KTP laser is in use, as the surgeon may decide to resect the tumor before using the laser.

2. Keep the TUR instrument set preferred by the surgeon nearby, including options for different resecting loops.

3. Make sure biopsy forceps, Bugbee fiber, and Bugbee cord are close by.

4. Confirm with the surgeon the type of fluid to hang:

   - Water and monopolar instrumentation are often more convenient for these procedures.

- Be prepared to switch to normal saline if bipolar instrumentation is required.

5. Be creative and innovative and adapt to any changes in the procedure as needed!

Transurethral Incision of Prostate/Bladder Neck (TUIP)

TUIP is a procedure aimed at reducing retrograde ejaculation caused by bladder neck issues in young men and facilitating better urine flow. The surgeon makes incisions at the bladder neck (the connection between the prostate and the bladder), typically at 5 o'clock and 7 o'clock positions.

This procedure can be performed using the TUR set, Direct Vision Internal Urethrotome (DVIU) set, or a laser, including the KTP laser. Based on this information, the following setup and equipment should be prepared.

<u>Preparation for the TUIP Procedure:</u>

- Pick and set up the default table.

- Have the following equipment available:

1. The TUR set (which may include the bipolar working element and cord).

2. The monopolar and bipolar energy generators.

3. Hot monopolar and bipolar knives.

4. Monopolar and bipolar #24 loop.

5. Patient grounding pad (grounding the patient is wise in case the procedure changes or monopolar is used).

6. 3000 ml of water and normal saline (depending on what set the healthcare provider uses).

7. A guide wire.

8. Council Foley catheters in sizes 16 Fr, 18 Fr, and 20 Fr or have different options for the Foley catheter.

9. 10cc syringe.

10. Vanburen sounds and/or other urethral dilators for different options.

11. Surgical gel or 2% uro-jet lidocaine.

12. Don't forget to place the foot pedal of the energy generator used by the surgeon near their foot.

If Plasma Cutting Loop and Button Is Used

1. Switch to the plasma energy generator.

2. Add the Button TUR set.

3. Add the loop, knife, and cord (as requested by the surgeon), and have the button available.

4. Hang normal saline.

5. Don't forget to place the foot pedal by the surgeon's foot.

If The KTP Laser Is Used

- Be aware of and have available equipment and supplies for the KTP Laser (Potassium Titanyl Phosphate Crystal).

- Follow laser regulations:

  1. Make sure laser signs are on doors.

  2. Have goggles available by the doors for anyone about to enter the room, and make sure there are goggles in the room for everyone, including the patient.

  3. Cover windows to protect against laser exposure.

  4. Have at least 1000 ml of water on the default table.

  5. Follow all other hospital laser regulations.

- Add the #17 resectoscope sheath and/or the laser sheath (used with the cystoscopy set).

- Add the laser fiber (200, 400, or 600, depending on the size preferred).

- Add the greenlight scope or a lens filter (obtained from the laser sales representative).

- Have the laser guide catheter or an open-ended catheter available (such as a Tigger Tail).

- Add a laser fiber holding device or use a wet towel to assist with holding the laser fiber.

Notes:

- When using a monopolar hot knife, set the energy generator to 70 cut and 70 coag. If the setting is increased, the knife may break during the procedure.

- For the TUIP, the KTP laser fiber (600 or 400) works better for this particular operation.

Cystoscopy Clot Evacuation

What Is It?

This procedure involves inspecting the urethra, bladder, ureters, and kidneys. In many cases, patients arrive in the operating room with a Foley catheter already inserted into the bladder, which may be filled with blood and clots. Therefore, visualization of the mentioned areas is necessary, followed by suctioning of the clots and, if needed, biopsy and removal of abnormal tissue using heat diathermy or laser.

Case Set Up

Be open-minded when setting up for this case. Visualize where the bleeding might originate. It's helpful if the urologist informs you of the specific needs for the procedure, but regardless, prepare creatively and have all potential items ready. For example:

- The default table

- A Toomey or Ellik evacuator

- Biopsy forceps (for use with the rigid cystoscope)

- Bugbee cord

- Bugbee electrode

- The transurethral resectoscope (monopolar or bipolar; check the doctor's preference)

- Loop electrodes for both monopolar and bipolar sets (make sure you have the appropriate electrode cord)

- Specimen cups

- Surgical lubricant or uro-jet

- Various Foley catheters, especially three-way options

- Foley bag or leg bag

- Statlock

- Continuous irrigation fluid (water, normal saline, or glycine)

- Be prepared to set up continuous bladder irrigation if needed

- Be ready for ureteroscopy if necessary (refer to ureteroscopy setup above)

The case may start as a simple in-and-out

procedure but could turn into a bladder biopsy/TURBT, TURP, ureteroscopy, stent placement, lithotripsy, or just a stent and/or Foley placement. The goal is to be ready for anything, from simple to complex. The key steps are to visualize, find the bleeding source, and stop it. Before the patient leaves the operating room, make sure the Foley catheter (if placed) is draining better than 'a little red,' as a great friend doctor says whenever he finishes the TURP procedures!

Cystolitholapaxy

What Is It?

Let's make it simple! 'Cysto' means bladder, 'litho' means stone, and 'lapa' refers to the abdomen. Cystolitholapaxy is a procedure to break up bladder stones and remove them. This can be achieved by manually crushing the stones with an instrument, using laser, ultrasound waves, graspers, baskets, or even gravity through a cystoscope sheath. Often, the procedure is performed through a cystoscope sheath with a Toomey or Ellik bladder evacuator. If the stone(s) are too large, an open abdominal procedure such as a cystostomy may be required.

Knowing these details, let's prepare for the procedure:

- Set up the case as a simple cystoscopic procedure, beginning with the default table.

- Have a stone grasper (if not already included in the cystoscopy set) and a disposable basket on hand (the stronger, the better, such as a 3.4 size).

- Make sure the stone crusher is available (though it can be a dangerous instrument).

- Prepare both a Toomey and an Ellik evacuator.

- Have a large basin for water (if using the Ellik).

- Larger cystoscopy sheaths (25 Fr.) and/or a TUR set should be ready.

- Make sure to have loops available - #24 and #26.

- Prepare the laser, laser key, and fibers (a 1,000 size is ideal or the largest fiber available for the specific laser being used).

- Know the location of the ultrasonic lithotripter equipment in case the provider opts for that method. If used, make sure you have a suction machine, two suction tubes, and a mucus specimen trap (if needed).

- Add a nephroscope for the ultrasonic lithotripter technique.

- It's advantageous to ground the patient.

- Hang water for better visibility and conductivity if necessary.

- Remember to place the foot pedals where the surgeon can easily access them with their feet.

Notes:

1. This procedure is usually performed in a regular cystoscopy room. If the stone is too large and the surgeon opts for an abdominal incision, the patient may be transferred to a different surgical room.

2. In case of an abdominal incision, follow the surgeon's preference card and hospital protocols. I hope to cover such abdominal interventions in future volumes.

3. Have a variety of Foley catheter options available, along with a Foley or leg bag, in case the surgeon decides to place one at the end of the case.

Nephrolithotomy

Although this procedure is typically approached from the back, I am including it here because lenses and continuous irrigation are used to visualize the stones for treatment. In addition, many radiologists (who usually create the initial kidney access with wires and nephrostomy tubes) require cystoscopic placement of an open-ended catheter in the affected ureter to inject Omnipaque during their part of the procedure. Therefore, I will divide this procedure into three parts:

Part I - Cystoscopy Open-Ended Catheter Placement

The cystoscopy portion is similar to the procedures mentioned above:

- Set up the 'default table.'

- Add: Omnipaque, an open-ended catheter, a 60cc syringe, catheter extension tubing, and a guide wire.

- Prepare the Foley catheter of the doctor's preference (usually 16 Fr), a urine bag, and something to secure the open-ended catheter to the Foley, such as umbilical tape, heavy suture, Steri-Strips, or tape.

- Include a uro-jet or lubricant gel.

- Place water on the table and hang a 3000 water bag as continuous irrigation.

Part II - Nephrostomy Tube/Access Insertion

The nephrostomy tube insertion is typically performed by the Interventional Radiology (IR) team. This can occur in the radiology department or a room equipped with all the necessary tools for the entire procedure. Make sure that the operating room has a 220-volt outlet available for the laser machine if needed. The nephrostomy tube may be placed on the same day as the nephrolithotomy, or the nephrostomy tube may be inserted one day and the nephrolithotomy performed at a later time. When this happens, a cystoscopy may not be necessary. The urologist performs the nephrolithotomy by inserting a safety wire, followed by the nephrostomy balloon, and finally, the access sheath.

If the urology team is involved with the IR portion, they are often present to assist in positioning the patient and providing equipment and supplies that the IR team may not have. The urologist is frequently present to verify that the access is correctly positioned for successful stone extraction.

For this part, it is wise to have a separate sterile table with the following:

- Prepping agent

- Towels and the main adhesive skin drape with a fluid collector and drain

- Instruments such as hemostats, scissors, a needle driver, and a knife

- Spinal needle

- Amplax guide wires (straight and angled glide)

- A bowl of water, N/S, Omnipaque, and local anesthetic injection

- Various milliliter syringes

- Dual-lumen catheter

- Open-ended catheter, pigtail catheter, or one based on the doctor's preference

- Fluoroscopy covers

- Suction tubing

- Other necessary items

Part III – Nephrolithotomy

It is very important to have a comprehensive list of all possible equipment and supplies for this procedure. Think of the big picture: consider the operating room setup, the operating table, patient positioning, operating side, equipment, wall outlets, extension cords, x-ray machine, suctions, and other essential elements. Ask important questions, such as: Is the operating room appropriate for this procedure? Where and how will the equipment be placed? Are there any special equipment needs? Is a sales representative available? Pay attention to the operating side, surgeon preferences, and specific requests.

Now, let's create a detailed list:

Equipment:

- Cysto table

- SCU machine

- Extension cord

- Fluid pole

- Perc cart (with extra supplies)

- X-ray lead

- Lithotripsy machine, equipment, and supplies

- Laser machine

- Camera/video tower

- Suction machine

- Transport monitor (if needed)

Note: Make sure an anesthesia cart is available before the procedure begins.

Positioning:

- Egg crate or foam

- Prone view

- Blue arm foam

- 4-6 pillows

- Orange gel chest rolls

- Safety strap

Instruments:

- Camera

- Flexible cystoscope

- Digital ureteroscope

- Lithotripsy supplies

- Perc neph tray

- Other lithotripsy equipment and supplies

Medications:

- Omnipaque

- Bottle of water (1000 ml)

- 3000 ml saline bags (x10)

- 1000 ml LR for anesthesia

- Urojet (2% lidocaine jelly)

- Local anesthetic agent (if needed)

Supplies:

- Extra-long suction tubing (x2)

- Ioban drape pouch (#6619, typically found in ortho core)

- Perc stone graspers

- Upper body Bair Hugger (make sure blankets are available)

- Laser fibers (200, 272, 365)

Note: Some surgeons may perform the cystoscopy on a

stretcher or in the cysto room. Administer antibiotics before going to Interventional Radiology. The video tower should be in the interventional radiology room to begin the cystoscopy on the stretcher.

Other Possible Needs

- Extra Nephromax balloon dilator (30 Fr.) and pressure device

- Amplax nephrostomy dilator set (sometimes required)

- 2nd cysto table

- 2nd gown and gloves

- An extra guide wire (especially Amplax, glide, and angle glide)

- 2nd flexible cystoscope

- 2nd Urojet (2% lidocaine jelly)

- 2nd cystoscopy camera

- 2nd cysto pack

- 2nd cysto tubing

- Flexible cystoscope graspers

- Extension tubing

- Open-ended catheters

- Umbilical tape

- Foley kit and Betadine prep sticks

- Various sizes of council tip Foley catheters (16, 18, 20, and 22)

- Open-ended ureteral catheters

- Piston syringe and extra 10cc syringes

- Different sizes of J-stents (e.g., 6x24, 6x26, and 6x28) – always verify with the doctor's preference.

Suture

- 2-0 silk or nylon

- 4-0 Monocryl or Vicryl

Final Dressing and Accessories

- 4x4 sponges

- Abdominal pads (ABD)

- Various types of adhesive tape

- Ostomy bags

- Extra urine bag

- Other necessary accessories

Nephrolithotomy Part Procedure

This procedure may be simple (in and out), but it can also take a long time, make it difficult to maintain a clear image on the monitor, and require extensive N/S irrigation. Sometimes, it is performed with just a nephroscope and a grasper, but other times, it may involve a flexible cystoscope, digital or non-digital ureteroscope, or even a disposable ureteroscope. As a result, the procedure can be challenging and requires a competent team to ensure success.

Now, let's walk through the steps once the initial nephrostomy wire is in place:

1. A second wire is placed for safety to prevent losing access. A dual-lumen catheter is helpful for this step.

2. Once the second wire is in place (usually a stiff or Amplatz wire), the NephroMax balloon is introduced to dilate the nephrostomy tract. Pressure is applied using a pressure device filled with Omnipaque.

3. After the tract is dilated, the nephrostomy access sheath is inserted.

4. The balloon is then removed, and the nephroscope is inserted to begin lithotripsy and stone extraction.

5. Once the stone(s) are removed, the ureteral catheter placed during the cystoscopy is removed, and a J-stent is inserted through the nephrostomy access sheath. Flexible graspers may be needed to make sure the J-stent is properly positioned.

6. With the J-stent in place, a council-tip Foley catheter is inserted. Some surgeons also prefer to insert an open-ended catheter for additional safety and access. To visualize the Foley, inflate its balloon using a 10cc syringe with a small amount of Omnipaque. A piston syringe filled with contrast can also help visualize the Foley's function, ensuring it drains correctly.

7. Once the open-ended catheter and Foley are inserted, secure them with a 2-0 suture (silk or nylon).

8. At this point, all wires can be safely removed, and the final dressing is applied: Foley or urostomy bag, 4x4 sponges, ABD pads, tape, etc.

9. The case is complete; the surgeon debriefs, and the team assists in transferring the patient to the stretcher.

UroLift

<u>What Is It?</u>

UroLift involves the insertion of tiny implants (clips) into the urethra to create space by holding enlarged prostate tissue away. This helps prevent urethral blockage and improves urine flow. The procedure is minimally invasive, requiring no cutting, tissue removal, or use of heat. Simply prepare the standard cystoscopy table. Typically, a UroLift company representative will provide a specialized 2.0 mm cystoscope and the pliers for inserting the clips, usually four.

HoLEP

HoLEP, or Holmium Laser Enucleation of the Prostate, is a minimally invasive procedure that uses pulses of a laser beam to remove tissue from inside the prostate. This creates more space for the urethra and improves urine flow.

<u>How to Set Up the Cystoscopy Table for HoLEP?</u>

- Prepare the standard cystoscopy table.

- Make sure a cystoscopy set is available.

- Add a nephroscope.

- Have a TURP set ready.

- Include a morcellator to remove the inner prostatic tissue once released. Be sure to include the morcellator blade.

- Make sure a nerve hook is available in one of your instrument sets, as it may be needed to unplug the morcellator.

- Bring the special morcellator machine into the operating room to serve as the energy source.

- Provide the laser fiber (550).

- Include a laser fiber access sheath for better laser fiber control.

- Make sure Van Buren sounds, and enough surgical gel are available.

- Have a 20-24 Fr three-way Foley catheter, a Foley bag, and normal saline for continuous bladder irrigation.

Conclusion

As I've said before, "I love urology!" It's my passion. If I had to choose one word to describe myself as a urology technologist, it would be 'innovation.' I love experimenting and finding better ways to do things. Sometimes, I tweak existing techniques or come up with new ideas, even if they seem like 'the same old ones.'

Let me conclude with two stories:

Case Scenario One

Three years ago, a urologist was performing a ureteroscopy with a resident. This doctor didn't like using contrast at the start of the case or inserting anything besides the wire and ureteroscope into the ureter. I wasn't the tech in that room, but I stopped by to see why the procedure was taking so long.

When I looked at the X-ray screen, I saw the wire was already in the kidney, and the doctors were struggling to pass the ureteroscope up the ureter. The stone was clearly visible next to the wire.

I asked, "What are you doing?"

They replied, "We've been trying to pass the ureteroscope into the kidney, but we can't."

I suggested, "The wire's already in place. Why don't you use an access sheath?"

They paused, looked at each other, and then at me, saying, "Good idea! Let's try it."

Long story short, they used the sheath, passed the ureteroscope, and successfully pulverized the stone. What I considered an 'old' idea turned out to be a new solution for them.

The next day, I received an email from my supervisor praising my innovative thinking. Shortly after, I received letters from the Urology Department Director and even the hospital CEO recognizing my contribution. I was very grateful.

Case Scenario Two

This case involved a patient in his 60s with an obstructed right distal ureter. He came into the room with a nephrostomy tube in place. During the cystoscopy, the urologist found the left ureteral orifice but couldn't locate the right one.

Since the nephrostomy tube was already in place, I suggested injecting contrast through it, followed by a guide wire. After we inserted the wire, its tip passed through the distal portion of the ureter, becoming visible in the bladder. I then recommended using the TUR set and a #24 loop to cut the ureteral orifice. Once the cut was made, the guide wire was visible, and the surgeon was able to pull it out through the urethra. A J-stent was placed, and the nephrostomy tube was removed.

The urologist was pleased with the unexpected solution and acknowledged my input. Unfortunately, the story didn't end as we hoped. When I saw the surgeon a few days later, he informed me the patient had refused dialysis and had passed away. We were both saddened by the outcome.

As a surgical urology team, we did our best, finding innovative ways to provide top-notch care for our patients. This edition is an effort to serve as a contemporary resource for helping the urology team anticipate both patient and surgeon needs, ensuring successful urologic endoscopic procedures.